The Complete Guide to Yoga:

Discovering Physical, Mental, and Spiritual Benefits of Yoga

by

Laura Trenaman

TABLE OF CONTENTS

INTRODUCTION

Yoga is a practice that originated in ancient India over 5,000 years ago. The word "yoga" comes from the Sanskrit word "yuj," which means to unite or yoke. It is a holistic practice that aims to integrate the mind, body, and spirit through physical postures, breathing techniques, meditation, and relaxation. There are many different types of yoga, each with its own focus and style. Yoga is often used for stress relief, relaxation, and to improve overall physical and mental health. Regular practice can improve flexibility, strength, balance, and posture, and also help reduce anxiety, depression, inflammation, chronic pain, and more. Yoga can be practiced by people of all ages and fitness levels, and is a powerful tool for cultivating self-awareness, mindfulness, and personal growth.

Yoga is thus a way of life. It teaches you to be in control of yourself and leads you on a path of honesty, making you a humble person. The best part about yoga is that it gives you the freedom to choose. So if you're someone who only wants to focus on physical well-being, you're totally allowed to do that. You can go about practicing your daily yoga routine without even bothering about the spiritual aspect of yoga and nobody will stop you. For whatever reason you decide to do yoga, yoga will definitely make you feel good about yourself.

Chapter 1:

CHOOSING THE RIGHT CLOTHES FOR YOGA

Choosing the right clothes for yoga is important to ensure comfort and ease of movement during practice. Here are some tips on how to choose the right clothes for yoga:

1. Choose clothes that are comfortable and non-restrictive. Yoga involves a lot of stretching and movement, so it is important to wear clothes that allow you to move freely.
2. Look for fabrics that are breathable and moisture-wicking. This will help keep you cool and dry during a sweaty yoga practice.
3. Consider the fit of your clothes. Clothing that is too tight may restrict movement, while clothing that is too loose may get in the way during certain poses. Look for clothes that fit well and allow for easy movement.
4. Choose clothes that are appropriate for the type of yoga you are practicing. For example, if you are practicing hot yoga, you may want to wear lighter weight clothing that is designed to wick away moisture.
5. Consider the length of your pants or shorts. If you are practicing a lot of inversions or standing poses, you may want to wear pants that are not too long and won't bunch up around your ankles.
6. Choose clothes that you feel comfortable and confident in. You want to be able to focus on your practice and not worry about your clothing.

Overall, the key to choosing the right clothes for yoga is to prioritize comfort, freedom of movement, and breathability. With the right clothing, you can fully focus on your practice and get the most out of your yoga session.

Chapter 2: YOGA SOCKS AND GLOVES

Yoga socks and gloves are specialized accessories that can be used during yoga practice. Here are some things to consider when deciding whether or not to use yoga socks and gloves:

1. Traction: Yoga socks and gloves are designed to provide traction, helping you to grip the mat and maintain stability during poses. If you find that you slip on your mat during certain poses, yoga socks or gloves may be helpful.
2. Hygiene: If you practice in a studio or gym, you may be concerned about the cleanliness of the shared mats. Yoga socks and gloves can provide a barrier between your skin and the mat, helping to reduce the risk of infection.
3. Comfort: Some people find that yoga socks and gloves provide additional comfort and support during practice, particularly if they have sensitive skin or experience discomfort in their hands or feet.
4. Cost: Yoga socks and gloves can be more expensive than regular socks and gloves, and may not be necessary for everyone. If you are on a budget, you may want to consider using regular socks or going barefoot during practice.
5. Style: Yoga socks and gloves come in a variety of styles and colors, and can be a fun way to express your personality and add some flair to your yoga practice.

Ultimately, whether or not to use yoga socks and gloves is a personal preference. Some people find them helpful for their practice, while others prefer to go barefoot or use regular socks and gloves. If you are considering purchasing yoga socks or gloves, it is important to choose a high-quality product that provides good traction and is comfortable to wear.

Chapter 3:
Choosing the Right Accessories and Props

Accessories and props can enhance your yoga practice by providing additional support, stability, and comfort. Here are some tips on how to choose the right accessories and props for your practice:

1. Consider your needs: Think about what you need to support your practice. For example, if you have tight hips, you may benefit from a bolster or yoga block to support your hips in seated poses.
2. Quality: Choose high-quality accessories and props that are durable and will last a long time. It is worth investing in quality products to ensure your safety and comfort during practice.
3. Size and shape: Make sure the size and shape of the accessory or prop fit your body and support your practice. For example, if you are using a yoga block, choose the appropriate height for your needs.
4. Material: Consider the material of the accessory or prop. For example, if you are using a yoga mat, choose a non-slip material that provides good traction.
5. Comfort: Choose accessories and props that are comfortable and feel good to use. You want to be able to focus on your practice and not be distracted by discomfort.
6. Cost: Accessories and props can be expensive, so consider your budget and choose products that provide the most value for your money.

Some common accessories and props for yoga include yoga blocks, straps, bolsters, blankets, and eye pillows. These props can be used to support your practice and help you achieve proper alignment in your poses. If you are unsure about which accessories and props to use, consider taking a class with a qualified instructor who can guide you through the use of these tools.

Chapter 4: EATING BEFORE PRACTICE

Eating before yoga practice can affect your performance and how you feel during the session. Here are some tips on how to eat before yoga practice:

1. Timing: It is recommended to wait for at least 2-3 hours after a large meal before practicing yoga. This allows your body to digest the food and prevents discomfort during practice. If you are hungry before practice, a light snack 30 minutes to an hour before can be beneficial.
2. Types of food: Avoid heavy, greasy, or spicy foods before practice as they can cause discomfort or digestive issues. Instead, choose light, easy-to-digest foods such as fruits, vegetables, and whole grains. You can also include some protein for sustained energy.
3. Hydration: Make sure to stay hydrated before, during, and after practice. Drink plenty of water throughout the day, and if you are practicing in a hot room or doing more intense practice, you may want to consider a sports drink or coconut water to replenish electrolytes.
4. Individual needs: Everyone's body is different, so pay attention to how you feel after eating before practice. Experiment with different types and timing of meals to find what works best for you.
5. Listen to your body: If you are feeling overly full or uncomfortable during practice, take a break and rest in the child's pose or other restorative poses. Don't push yourself to perform if you are feeling unwell.

Overall, it is important to be mindful of what you eat before yoga practice to ensure that you have enough energy to sustain your practice without causing discomfort or digestive issues. Be sure to listen to your body and make adjustments as needed.

Chapter 5: Arriving Early

Arriving early to your yoga class is a great way to prepare for your practice and get the most out of your session. Here are some benefits of arriving early:

1. Settle in: Arriving early allows you to settle in and get comfortable in the space. You can lay out your mat, adjust the lighting, and get familiar with your surroundings.
2. Connect with the teacher: Arriving early gives you the opportunity to connect with your yoga teacher before class. You can ask questions, express any concerns or injuries, and get personalized guidance.
3. Breathwork and meditation: Many yoga classes start with breathwork or meditation. Arriving early gives you time to prepare for this and get into the right headspace before class begins.
4. Warm-up: Arriving early also gives you time to do a quick warm-up before class begins. This can help prevent injuries and prepare your body for practice.
5. Mindfulness: Arriving early allows you to practice mindfulness and be present at the moment. You can use this time to focus on your breath, set an intention for your practice, or simply take a moment to relax and unwind.

Overall, arriving early to your yoga class can help you get the most out of your practice and prepare your body and mind for the session. It also allows you to connect with your teacher and get personalized guidance. Try arriving a few minutes early to your next yoga class and see how it affects your practice.

Chapter 6: PRACTICE, PRACTICE, PRACTICE

Yoga practice is the act of performing yoga postures or asanas in a focused and intentional manner. Yoga practice is typically performed on a yoga mat and involves a combination of physical postures, breathwork, meditation, and relaxation techniques.

Here are some tips for successful yoga practice:

1. Set an intention: Before beginning your practice, take a moment to set an intention. This can be anything from finding inner peace to increasing flexibility. Having a clear intention can help focus your mind and keep you motivated throughout your practice.
2. Warm-up: Begin your practice with a few gentle warm-up poses to prepare your body for more intense postures. This can help prevent injuries and make your practice more comfortable.
3. Proper alignment: Pay attention to proper alignment in each posture. This can help prevent injuries and increase the effectiveness of the pose.
4. Breathwork: Focus on your breath throughout your practice. Use your breath to help you stay present and connected to your body. Coordinate your breath with each movement and try to maintain smooth and even breathing.
5. Modify as needed: Don't be afraid to modify poses to suit your needs. Use props or modify postures to make them more accessible or comfortable for you. Listen to your body and make adjustments as needed.
6. End with relaxation: End your practice with a few minutes of relaxation or meditation. This can help calm your mind and reduce stress.

Remember that yoga is a practice, and it takes time and consistency to see progress. Be patient with yourself, and enjoy the journey. By focusing on proper alignment, breathwork, and relaxation, you can experience the many benefits of yoga practice, including increased strength, flexibility, and overall well-being.

Chapter 7: STYLES OF YOGA

There are many styles of yoga, each with its own unique focus and approach to the practice. Here are some of the most common styles of yoga:

1. **Hatha Yoga**: Hatha yoga is a gentle, slow-paced practice that emphasizes breathwork and basic postures. It is a good style for beginners or those looking for a more relaxed practice.
2. **Vinyasa Yoga**: Vinyasa yoga is a more dynamic style that links movement with breath. It typically involves flowing from one posture to the next in a sequence.
3. **Ashtanga Yoga**: Ashtanga yoga is a more physically demanding style that involves a set sequence of postures performed in a specific order. It is a good style for those looking for a more intense workout.
4. **Bikram Yoga**: Bikram yoga is a style of yoga practiced in a heated room, typically around 105°F. It involves a set sequence of 26 postures and two breathing exercises.
5. **Iyengar Yoga**: Iyengar yoga emphasizes proper alignment and uses props such as blocks, straps, and blankets to help students achieve correct alignment in each posture.
6. **Restorative Yoga**: Restorative yoga is a gentle style that involves holding postures for several minutes at a time. It is a good style for those looking to relax and release tension.
7. **Kundalini Yoga**: Kundalini yoga focuses on breathwork, meditation, and spiritual awareness. It involves a combination of physical postures, breathwork, and chanting.

8. **Yin Yoga**: Yin yoga is a slow-paced style that involves holding postures for several minutes at a time to stretch the connective tissues and increase flexibility.

These are just a few of the many styles of yoga available. It is important to find a style that resonates with you and your goals for your practice.

Hatha Yoga

Hatha yoga is a traditional style of yoga that focuses on physical postures (asanas), breathwork (pranayama), and meditation. It is one of the most widely practiced styles of yoga and is often recommended for beginners due to its slower pace and focus on basic postures.

Hatha yoga is a holistic practice that aims to balance the body, mind, and spirit. It is based on the idea that the body and mind are connected, and that physical postures can help bring balance to the entire system. In Hatha yoga, each posture is held for several breaths, allowing the body to release tension and increase flexibility.

Some of the benefits of practicing Hatha yoga include increased flexibility, strength, and balance; reduced stress and anxiety; improved digestion and circulation; and a greater sense of overall well-being.

Hatha yoga classes typically begin with a few minutes of centering and breathwork, followed by a series of physical postures that are held for several breaths each. Classes may also include seated meditation or relaxation at the end.

Hatha yoga can be practiced by people of all ages and fitness levels. It is a gentle and accessible style of yoga that can be adapted to suit individual needs and abilities.

Vinyasa Yoga

Vinyasa yoga is a style of yoga that emphasizes movement and breath, linking each posture to an inhale or exhale. It is a dynamic and flowing practice that is often described as a moving meditation.

In Vinyasa yoga, each posture is coordinated with the breath, creating a seamless flow of movement from one posture to the next. The pace of the practice can vary depending on the teacher and the level of the class, but it is typically faster than Hatha yoga and other more static styles.

The benefits of practicing Vinyasa yoga include increased strength, flexibility, and cardiovascular endurance; improved balance and coordination; reduced stress and anxiety; and a greater sense of mindfulness and relaxation.

Vinyasa yoga classes typically begin with a few minutes of centering and breathwork, followed by a series of dynamic postures that flow together in a sequence. The class may include a variety of standing, seated, and balancing postures, as well as inversions and backbends. Classes may also include pranayama (breathing exercises), meditation, or relaxation at the end.

Vinyasa yoga can be challenging, but it is suitable for people of all ages and fitness levels. Modifications and variations of postures are often offered to accommodate different abilities and needs.

Ashtanga Yoga

Ashtanga yoga is a physically demanding style of yoga that involves a set sequence of postures performed in a specific order. It is a dynamic and athletic practice that focuses on building strength, flexibility, and endurance.

The Ashtanga yoga system consists of six series of postures, each with a specific focus and level of difficulty. The first series, known as the Primary Series, is the foundation of the practice and includes a sequence of standing, seated, and finishing postures. Each posture is linked to an inhale or exhale, creating a continuous flow of movement.

Ashtanga yoga is traditionally practiced as a self-led practice, with students memorizing the sequence of postures and moving through the sequence at their own pace. However, many Ashtanga yoga classes are now led by teachers, with students following the teacher's guidance and moving through the sequence together.

The benefits of practicing Ashtanga yoga include increased strength, flexibility, and endurance; improved focus and concentration; and a greater sense of overall well-being.

Ashtanga yoga can be challenging, and it is recommended for those with some prior yoga experience. It is a good choice for those looking for a more athletic and physically demanding practice. However, modifications and variations of postures are often offered to accommodate different abilities and needs.

Bikram Yoga

Bikram yoga, also known as hot yoga, is a style of yoga that is practiced in a heated room. The practice consists of a set sequence of 26 postures and two breathing exercises, and the room is typically heated to around 105°F (40°C) with a humidity of 40%.

The heat in Bikram yoga is believed to help facilitate deeper stretching and detoxification through sweating. The practice also aims to improve cardiovascular health, increase strength and flexibility, and reduce stress and anxiety.

Bikram yoga classes are typically 90 minutes long and follow the same sequence of postures and breathing exercises each time. The sequence is designed to work all parts of the body, with a focus on the spine, muscles, and joints.

Bikram yoga can be challenging due to the heat and intensity of the practice. It is not recommended for everyone, particularly those with certain medical conditions or who are sensitive to heat. It is important to stay well-hydrated and listen to your body during Bikram yoga classes.

Some people find the heat and intensity of Bikram yoga to be invigorating and beneficial for their physical and mental health, while others prefer a cooler and gentler style of yoga. It is important to choose a yoga style that feels right for your body and your goals.

Iyengar Yoga

Iyengar yoga is a style of yoga that emphasizes precision, alignment, and the use of props to support the body in postures. It was developed by B.K.S. Iyengar, who is widely regarded as one of the foremost yoga teachers of the modern era.

In Iyengar yoga, the focus is on developing strength, flexibility, and balance while maintaining proper alignment in each posture. The use of props such as blocks, straps, and blankets is encouraged to help students achieve correct alignment and deepen their practice.

Iyengar yoga classes typically begin with a few minutes of centering and breathwork, followed by a series of standing, seated, and reclining postures. The pace of the practice is generally slower than other styles of yoga, with an emphasis on holding each posture for longer periods.

The benefits of practicing Iyengar yoga include increased strength, flexibility, and balance; improved posture and alignment; reduced stress and anxiety; and a greater sense of mindfulness and relaxation.

Iyengar yoga is suitable for people of all ages and fitness levels, and modifications and variations of postures are often offered to accommodate different abilities and needs. It is a good choice for those who are interested in developing a strong foundation in yoga and who appreciate the attention to detail and alignment in their practice.

Restorative Yoga

Restorative yoga is a gentle and relaxing style of yoga that uses props to support the body in comfortable, passive poses. The focus is on slowing down, releasing the tension, and promoting deep relaxation.

Restorative yoga poses are designed to help the body and mind release tension and stress. The use of props such as blankets, bolsters, and blocks allows the body to fully relax into each pose, and the longer holds of each pose allow the mind to be calm and quiet.

Restorative yoga can be especially beneficial for people who are experiencing stress, anxiety, or fatigue, as well as those recovering from illness or injury. It can also be a good choice for those who are new to yoga or who are looking for a gentle, calming practice.

During a restorative yoga class, students typically move through a series of poses, holding each pose for several minutes at a time. The focus is on deep breathing and releasing the tension, rather than on building strength or flexibility.

The benefits of practicing restorative yoga include reduced stress and anxiety, improved sleep quality, increased flexibility and range of motion, and a greater sense of overall well-being.

Restorative yoga is suitable for people of all ages and fitness levels, and modifications and variations of poses can be offered to accommodate different abilities and needs. It is a good choice for anyone looking to slow down, relax, and rejuvenate their body and mind.

Kundalini Yoga

Kundalini yoga is a style of yoga that focuses on the awakening of the "kundalini energy," which is said to be coiled at the base of the spine. This energy is believed to be a source of spiritual and creative power, and the practice of Kundalini yoga is designed to help it rise through the chakras, or energy centers, of the body.

Kundalini yoga classes typically involve a combination of physical postures, breathwork, chanting, and meditation. The postures are often repetitive and dynamic, and the focus is on moving energy through the body and awakening the kundalini energy.

The practice of Kundalini yoga can be intense and transformative, and it is said to offer a range of benefits for the body, mind, and spirit. These benefits may include increased energy and vitality, improved physical and mental health, heightened creativity and intuition, and a greater sense of spiritual connection.

Kundalini yoga is suitable for people of all ages and fitness levels, and modifications and variations of postures can be offered to accommodate different abilities and needs. It is a good choice for those who are interested in exploring the spiritual and energetic dimensions of yoga, as well as those who are looking for a challenging and transformative practice.

Yin Yoga

Yin yoga is a slow, meditative style of yoga that focuses on stretching and lengthening the connective tissues in the body, such as the ligaments, tendons, and fascia. This is done through a series of seated or reclined poses that are held for several minutes at a time.

The goal of yin yoga is to increase flexibility and joint mobility, as well as to promote relaxation and mindfulness. By holding the poses for longer periods of time, students are encouraged to tune into their bodies and their breath and to develop a greater sense of inner stillness and awareness.

Yin yoga can be a good choice for people who are looking to complement a more active, yang-style yoga practice or who are looking for a gentler, more meditative form of exercise. It is also a good choice for those who are recovering from injury or illness, as the slow, supported poses can help to relieve tension and promote healing.

The benefits of practicing yin yoga include increased flexibility and joint mobility, improved circulation, reduced stress and anxiety, and a greater sense of overall well-being. It can be practiced by people of all ages and fitness levels, and modifications and variations of poses can be offered to accommodate different abilities and needs.

Hot Yoga

Hot yoga is a style of yoga that is practiced in a heated room, typically with temperatures ranging from 90 to 105 degrees Fahrenheit. The heat is used to increase flexibility, improve circulation, and promote detoxification through sweating.

There are several types of hot yoga, but the most well-known is Bikram yoga, which consists of a specific sequence of 26 postures and two breathing exercises that are practiced in a room heated to 105 degrees Fahrenheit with a humidity of 40%. Other styles of hot yoga may incorporate different postures and breathing exercises, but they are all typically practiced in a heated room.

The benefits of practicing hot yoga may include increased flexibility, improved cardiovascular health, reduced stress and anxiety, and enhanced detoxification. However, practicing yoga in a hot environment can also pose risks, particularly for people with certain health conditions, such as high blood pressure or heart problems. It is important to consult with a healthcare provider before beginning a hot yoga practice to listen to your body and take breaks as needed during class.

If you are interested in trying hot yoga, it is important to come to class prepared by staying hydrated, wearing lightweight and breathable clothing, and bringing a towel and water bottle. Additionally, it is recommended to start with a beginner-level class and to communicate with the instructor if you have any concerns or questions.

Prenatal Yoga

Prenatal yoga is a type of yoga that is specifically designed for pregnant women. It can help expectant mothers to stay active, relieve stress, and prepare their bodies for childbirth.

Prenatal yoga classes typically focus on gentle, low-impact exercises that help to strengthen the muscles that are important for labor and delivery, such as the pelvic floor muscles and the abdominal muscles. The classes also incorporate breathing techniques and relaxation exercises that can help to reduce stress and anxiety and promote a sense of calm.

In addition to the physical benefits, prenatal yoga can also help expectant mothers to connect with their growing babies and prepare mentally and emotionally for the challenges of childbirth and motherhood. It can also be a great way to connect with other expectant mothers and build a supportive community.

When practicing prenatal yoga, it is important to work with a qualified instructor who has experience working with pregnant women. The instructor can help to modify poses and movements as needed to accommodate the changing needs and abilities of expectant mothers.

It is also important to listen to your body and avoid any poses or movements that feel uncomfortable or cause pain. Pregnant women should also consult with their healthcare provider before beginning a prenatal yoga practice to ensure that it is safe for them and their growing baby.

Tadasana

Tadasana, also known as Mountain Pose, is a foundational yoga posture that is often used as a starting point for other standing poses. It is a simple yet powerful pose that can help to improve posture, balance, and concentration.

To practice Tadasana, stand with your feet hip-distance apart and parallel to each other. Press down evenly through all four corners of your feet, and engage your leg muscles to lift your kneecaps and firm your thighs. Draw your tailbone down towards the floor to lengthen your lower back, and lift the crown of your head towards the ceiling to lengthen your spine.

Roll your shoulders back and down, and extend your arms alongside your body with your palms facing forward. Relax your facial muscles, and focus your gaze softly ahead of you.

In Tadasana, the body should be aligned and active, yet relaxed and grounded. It is a great pose for improving overall posture and body awareness and can be practiced at any time throughout the day to help bring a sense of grounding and stability.

Tadasana is also often used as a starting point for other standing poses, such as Warrior I and II, as well as for balancing poses such as Tree Pose. It is a foundational posture that can help to improve overall alignment and stability in the body, both on and off the mat.

Uttanasana

Uttanasana, also known as Standing Forward Bend, is a yoga pose that involves folding the torso forward and bending at the hips while standing. It is a simple yet powerful pose that can help to stretch the hamstrings, calves, and lower back, as well as calm the mind and relieve stress.

To practice Uttanasana, stand with your feet hip-distance apart and parallel to each other. Inhale and lift your arms overhead, lengthening your spine. Exhale and fold forward from the hips, keeping your knees slightly bent as needed to protect your lower back.

As you fold forward, allow your head and neck to release towards the ground, and let your arms and hands hang down towards the floor. If possible, bring your hands to the ground on either side of your feet, or hold onto your shins or ankles.

In Uttanasana, the focus is on folding forward and releasing tension in the back of the body, rather than on achieving a specific depth of the pose. It is important to listen to your body and avoid any pain or discomfort.

Uttanasana can be practiced on its own as a gentle stretch or as part of a larger yoga sequence. It is a great pose to practice anytime you need to release tension or calm the mind and can be especially beneficial for people who spend a lot of time sitting or standing in one position.

Dandasana

Dandasana, also known as Staff Pose, is a seated yoga posture that involves sitting with the legs extended forward and the spine upright. It is a foundational pose that can help to improve posture, strengthen the back muscles, and calm the mind.

To practice Dandasana, begin by sitting on the floor with your legs extended forward and your hands resting on the floor beside your hips. Press down through your sitting bones and engage your leg muscles to lift your kneecaps and firm your thighs.

Lengthen your spine upward and draw your shoulder blades down your back. Keep your chest open and your chin parallel to the floor. If you have tight hamstrings or lower back pain, you can sit on a folded blanket or block to help lift your pelvis and release tension in the lower back.

In Dandasana, the focus is on sitting with a tall, upright spine and engaged legs. It can be challenging to maintain this posture for an extended period of time, but with practice, it can help to improve overall posture and body awareness.

Dandasana is often used as a starting point for other seated poses, such as Paschimottanasana (Seated Forward Bend) and Janu Sirsasana (Head-to-Knee Forward Bend). It can also be practiced on its own as a way to improve posture and build strength in the back muscles.

Virabhadrasana

Virabhadrasana, also known as Warrior Pose, is a standing yoga posture that involves stretching the arms and legs in opposite directions. It is a powerful pose that can help to build strength, balance, and focus.

To practice Virabhadrasana, begin by standing at the front of your mat with your feet hip-distance apart. Step your left foot back about 3-4 feet and turn it out slightly, while keeping your right foot facing forward. Square your hips towards the front of the mat.

Inhale and lift your arms overhead, reaching your fingertips towards the sky. Exhale and bend your right knee, keeping it directly over your ankle. Press down through the outer edge of your left foot and engage your left thigh.

Draw your shoulder blades down your back and lift your chest. Gaze forward or slightly upward, and hold the pose for several breaths. Repeat on the other side by stepping your right foot back and bending your left knee.

Virabhadrasana can be practiced on its own as a way to build strength and balance, or as part of a larger yoga sequence. It is a great pose to practice anytime you need to feel strong and grounded and can be especially beneficial for people who spend a lot of time sitting or standing in one position. Variations of the pose include Virabhadrasana II and III, which involve different leg and arm positions.

Paschimottanasana

Paschimottanasana, also known as Seated Forward Bend, is a seated yoga posture that involves bending forward from the hips to stretch the entire back of the body. It is a calming pose that can help to release tension in the back, hips, and hamstrings.

To practice Paschimottanasana, begin by sitting on the floor with your legs extended forward and your hands resting on the floor beside your hips. Inhale and reach your arms overhead, lengthening your spine. Exhale and hinge forward from your hips, reaching your hands towards your feet.

Keep your spine long and your chest opens as you fold forward. If you have tight hamstrings, you can bend your knees slightly or use a strap around your feet to help you reach forward. Hold the pose for several breaths, then release and come back up to a seated position.

Paschimottanasana can be practiced on its own as a way to stretch and release tension in the back of the body, or as part of a larger yoga sequence. It is a great pose to practice in the morning to help wake up the body, or in the evening to help relax and prepare for sleep.

Variations of the pose include Janu Sirsasana, which involves stretching one leg at a time, and Paschimottanasana with a Twist, which involves twisting the torso to one side to deepen the stretch. As with all yoga poses, it is important to listen to your body and modify the pose as needed to avoid injury.

Pawanmuktasana

Pawanmuktasana, also known as Wind-Relieving Pose, is a reclining yoga posture that involves bringing the knees into the chest to massage the digestive organs and release tension in the lower back.

To practice Pawanmuktasana, begin by lying flat on your back with your legs extended and your arms resting at your sides. Inhale and bring your right knee towards your chest, interlacing your fingers around your shin to hold the knee in place. Exhale and gently pull your knee towards your chest, keeping your left leg extended on the floor.

Hold the pose for several breaths, then release your right leg and repeat on the left side. Once you have practiced both sides, bring both knees towards your chest and hug them in towards your body, rocking gently from side to side to release tension in the lower back.

Pawanmuktasana can be practiced on its own as a way to release tension and improve digestion, or as part of a larger yoga sequence. It is a great pose to practice after meals or when you are feeling bloated or uncomfortable in the digestive area.

Variations of the pose include Double Leg Wind-Relieving Pose, which involves bringing both knees towards the chest at the same time, and Half Wind-Relieving Pose, which involves stretching one leg at a time while holding the other knee towards the chest. As with all yoga poses, it is important to listen to your body and modify the pose as needed to avoid injury.

Trikonasana

Trikonasana, also known as Triangle Pose, is a standing yoga posture that stretches and strengthens the legs, hips, and spine.

To practice Trikonasana, begin by standing with your feet hip-width apart and your arms extended out to the sides. Turn your right foot out to the side, keeping your left foot pointing forward. Inhale and reach your right arm towards the right side, lengthening your spine. Exhale and bend sideways from your hips, keeping your left arm pointing towards the ceiling.

Rest your right hand on your shin or ankle, or on a block placed next to your foot. Extend your left arm towards the ceiling, keeping your gaze directed towards your left hand. Hold the pose for several breaths, then release and repeat on the other side.

Variations of the pose include using a strap to help reach the hand to the floor or practicing the pose with the back against a wall for added stability. As with all yoga poses, it is important to listen to your body and modify the pose as needed to avoid injury.

Trikonasana is a great pose for improving balance and posture, and for stretching and strengthening the muscles of the legs, hips, and spine. It is often practiced as part of a larger yoga sequence or as a stand-alone posture.

Adho Mukha Svanasana

Adho Mukha Svanasana, also known as Downward-Facing Dog Pose, is a common yoga posture that stretches and strengthens the whole body, especially the arms, shoulders, hamstrings, calves, and spine.

To practice Adho Mukha Svanasana, begin on your hands and knees with your wrists under your shoulders and your knees under your hips. Spread your fingers wide and press into your palms, lifting your hips up towards the ceiling.

Straighten your arms and legs, coming into an inverted V-shape with your body. Press your heels towards the floor and lengthen your spine, drawing your shoulder blades down your back. Keep your head and neck relaxed.

Hold the pose for several breaths, then release and come back to your hands and knees. Adho Mukha Svanasana can be practiced on its own as a way to stretch and strengthen the body, or as part of a larger yoga sequence.

Variations of the pose include using blocks under your hands if your hamstrings are tight, or bending one knee and straightening the other to stretch one leg at a time. As with all yoga poses, it is important to listen to your body and modify the pose as needed to avoid injury.

Vrikshasana

Vrikshasana, also known as Tree Pose, is a standing yoga posture that develops balance, strength, and concentration. This pose mimics the steady and graceful stance of a tree, with the roots firmly planted into the ground.

To practice Vrikshasana, begin by standing with your feet hip-width apart and your arms by your sides. Shift your weight onto your left foot, and bring the sole of your right foot to rest on the inside of your left thigh. If this is challenging, you can place your foot on the inside of your left calf instead, avoiding the knee joint.

Press your right foot into your left thigh, and bring your hands to your heart in the prayer position. Lengthen your spine and draw your shoulder blades down your back. Focus on a point in front of you to help with balance. Hold the pose for several breaths, then release and repeat on the other side.

Variations of the pose include extending the arms overhead or bringing the foot to rest on the opposite shin or ankle. As with all yoga poses, it is important to listen to your body and modify the pose as needed to avoid injury.

Vrikshasana helps to improve balance and stability, strengthen the legs and core, and cultivate concentration and focus. It is often practiced as part of a larger yoga sequence or as a stand-alone posture.

Bhujangasana

Bhujangasana, also known as Cobra Pose, is a backbend posture in yoga that strengthens the spine, arms, and shoulders, and opens up the chest and lungs. This pose is named after the cobra, as the pose resembles the raised hood of a cobra.

To practice Bhujangasana, begin by lying face down on your mat with your hands placed palms down near your shoulders. Inhale and press your hands into the mat, lifting your head and chest off the ground. Keep your elbows close to your body and your shoulders relaxed.

Straighten your arms and lift your chest as high as you comfortably can. Keep your gaze forward and draw your shoulder blades down your back. Engage your core and press the tops of your feet into the ground.

Hold the pose for several breaths, then release and lower your chest and head back down to the mat. Bhujangasana can be practiced on its own as a way to stretch and strengthen the body, or as part of a larger yoga sequence.

Variations of the pose include lifting the hands off the mat, bending the elbows, and bringing the hands further back towards the hips to deepen the stretch. As with all yoga poses, it is important to listen to your body and modify the pose as needed to avoid injury.

Marjariasana and Bitilasana

Marjariasana and Bitilasana are two yoga postures often practiced together as a gentle warm-up for the spine. They are also known as Cat Pose and Cow Pose, respectively.

To practice Marjariasana or Cat Pose, start on your hands and knees with your wrists directly under your shoulders and your knees under your hips. Inhale and arch your back, lifting your tailbone and head towards the ceiling. Draw your shoulders away from your ears.

On the exhale, round your spine, dropping your head towards the ground and tucking your chin to your chest. Draw your navel towards your spine and engage your core.

To practice Bitilasana or Cow Pose, begin in the same position as Marjariasana. On the inhale, lift your head and tailbone towards the ceiling, arching your back and dropping your belly towards the ground. Draw your shoulders away from your ears.

On the exhale, come back to Marjariasana or Cat Pose, rounding your spine and dropping your head towards the ground.

You can move back and forth between these two postures several times, syncing your breath with the movement. Marjariasana and Bitilasana can help to stretch and warm up the spine, improve circulation, and release tension in the neck and shoulders.

Malasana

Malasana, also known as Garland Pose or Yogic Squat, is a yoga posture that involves squatting down with your feet close together and your arms stretched forward. It is a great pose to stretch your hips, lower back, and thighs, and to increase flexibility and strength in your lower body.

To practice Malasana, begin by standing with your feet hip-distance apart. Slowly bend your knees and lower your hips down towards the ground, keeping your feet close together and your heels on the floor. Bring your hands together in front of your chest and press your elbows against the inner part of your knees, pushing them apart.

If it's challenging for you to keep your heels on the ground, you can place a folded blanket or a block underneath them. You can also use your elbows to press your knees outwards gently.

Once you find a comfortable position, stretch your arms forward and try to lengthen your spine, keeping your neck in line with your spine. You can hold this pose for several breaths, gradually increasing the time as you become more comfortable.

Malasana is a great pose to practice if you spend a lot of time sitting or if you want to improve your balance and flexibility. It can also help to improve digestion and stimulate the abdominal organs.

Balasana

Balasana, also known as Child's Pose, is a restorative yoga posture that is often used as a resting pose during a yoga practice. It is a gentle and relaxing pose that can help to calm the mind and relieve stress and tension in the body.

To practice Balasana, begin on your hands and knees, with your hands shoulder-width apart and your knees hip-width apart. Slowly lower your hips down towards your heels and rest your forehead on the ground, stretching your arms forward with your palms facing down.

If you find it difficult to rest your forehead on the ground, you can place a blanket or a block underneath your forehead to make yourself more comfortable.

Once you are in the pose, take several deep breaths, focusing on your breath and allowing your body to relax and release tension. You can stay in this pose for several breaths or several minutes, depending on your comfort level.

Balasana is a great pose to practice if you are feeling stressed, anxious, or overwhelmed, as it can help to calm the mind and soothe the nervous system. It can also help to stretch the hips, thighs, and ankles and relieve tension in the back, neck, and shoulders.

Setu Bandhasana

Setu Bandhasana, also known as Bridge Pose, is a yoga posture that is often used to stretch and strengthen the back, hips, and legs.

To practice Setu Bandhasana, begin by lying flat on your back with your knees bent and your feet flat on the ground, hip-width apart. Your arms should be resting by your sides with your palms facing down.

Next, slowly lift your hips up towards the ceiling, pressing down into your feet and engaging your glutes and hamstrings. Keep your shoulders and head on the ground, and hold the pose for several breaths.

If you feel comfortable in the pose, you can interlace your fingers underneath your back and press your arms and shoulders into the ground to deepen the stretch.

To release the pose, slowly lower your hips back down to the ground and release your arms by your sides.

Setu Bandhasana can help to improve flexibility and strengthen the muscles of the back, hips, and legs. It can also help to alleviate back pain and relieve tension in the neck and shoulders. Additionally, it can help to calm the mind and reduce stress and anxiety.

Baddha Konasana

Baddha Konasana, also known as Bound Angle Pose or Butterfly Pose, is a seated yoga posture that is commonly used to stretch the hips, thighs, and groin.

To practice Baddha Konasana, begin by sitting on the ground with your legs extended in front of you. Bend your knees and bring the soles of your feet together, allowing your knees to fall out to the sides.

Using your hands, gently grasp your ankles or feet and draw them in towards your pelvis. Lengthen your spine and sit up tall, engaging your core muscles.

If you feel comfortable in the pose, you can gently begin to fold forward, keeping your spine long and your chest lifted. You can rest your hands on your feet, ankles, or the ground in front of you.

Hold the pose for several breaths, and then slowly release the stretch and return to a seated position.

Baddha Konasana can help to improve flexibility in the hips, thighs, and groin, and can also help to alleviate menstrual cramps and symptoms of menopause. Additionally, it can help to stimulate the abdominal organs and improve digestion and can help to calm the mind and reduce stress and anxiety.

Supta Matsyendrasana

Supta Matsyendrasana, also known as Supine Spinal Twist or Reclining Twist, is a yoga pose that helps to stretch the muscles of the back, hips, and legs, while also providing a gentle massage to the internal organs.

To practice Supta Matsyendrasana, begin by lying on your back with your legs extended and your arms at your sides. Bend your right knee and bring it towards your chest, keeping your left leg extended.

Exhale and draw your right knee across your body towards the left side of your mat, twisting your torso to the right. You can keep your right arm extended out to the side or bring it into a T-shape with your left arm.

Gaze over your right shoulder and breathe deeply, feeling the stretch in your spine, hips, and inner thighs. Hold the pose for several breaths, and then release and repeat on the other side.

Supta Matsyendrasana can help to improve spinal mobility, relieve tension in the back and hips, and stimulate digestion. It can also help to calm the mind and reduce stress and anxiety. It is important to avoid forcing the twist and to listen to your body's limitations.

Savasana

Savasana, also known as Corpse Pose, is a yoga pose that is typically practiced at the end of a yoga session to help relax and rejuvenate the body and mind.

To practice Savasana, begin by lying on your back with your legs and arms extended, palms facing up. Close your eyes and allow your body to relax completely, letting go of any tension in your muscles.

Focus on your breath, inhaling deeply through your nose and exhaling slowly through your mouth. Let go of any thoughts or distractions and simply be present at the moment.

Savasana can be practiced for a few minutes or for as long as you like, and it is an essential part of any yoga practice. It helps to reduce stress, lower blood pressure, and improve sleep quality. It is important to ensure that you are comfortable and warm during Savasana and to allow yourself to completely surrender to the pose.

Chapter 8:

The Importance of Flexibility in a Successful Yoga Practice

Flexibility is a key component of successful yoga practice, as it enables you to move more freely and deeply into each pose. However, it is important to remember that flexibility is not the only goal of yoga. Yoga also emphasizes strength, balance, and mindfulness, all of which are essential for a healthy and balanced body and mind.

There are many different factors that can impact your flexibility, including age, genetics, injury history, and daily habits. While some people may naturally be more flexible than others, everyone can benefit from incorporating regular stretching and yoga practice into their routine.

It is important to remember that flexibility is not something that can be achieved overnight, but rather is a gradual process that requires consistent practice and patience. It is also important to approach flexibility training with care and to avoid pushing your body beyond its limits, which can lead to injury.

Overall, while flexibility is an important aspect of yoga, it is just one piece of the puzzle. A balanced yoga practice will focus on developing strength, flexibility, balance, and mindfulness in equal measure, in order to support your overall health and well-being.

Chapter 9:

Yoga is for People of All Shapes and Sizes

This statement is a common misconception about yoga. Yoga is a practice that can be adapted to suit people of all shapes, sizes, and fitness levels. While many people who practice yoga may be slender, this is not a requirement for practicing yoga or for experiencing the benefits of the practice.

Yoga is not just about physical fitness or achieving a certain body type. Rather, it is a holistic practice that encompasses physical movement, breath work, mindfulness, and meditation. Yoga can be a tool for promoting physical health and fitness, as well as mental and emotional well-being.

In fact, many yoga classes and studios have embraced a more inclusive approach to yoga, offering classes that cater to people of all shapes and sizes, and promoting body positivity and self-acceptance. Additionally, there are many online resources and videos available that offer modifications and adaptations for different body types and abilities.

Ultimately, yoga is a practice that is accessible to everyone, regardless of their size or shape. It is important to remember that yoga is not about achieving a certain physical ideal, but rather about cultivating a healthy and balanced body and mind through mindful movement and breath work.

Chapter 10:

Common Misconceptions about Practicing Yoga

This statement is another common misconception about yoga. While there are certain yoga postures that may not be comfortable or beneficial during menstruation, yoga can actually be a helpful tool for managing menstrual cramps, mood swings, and other symptoms associated with periods.

Gentle yoga postures such as forward fold, gentle twists, and supported restorative poses can help to alleviate cramps and discomfort, while relaxation and breathing techniques can help to reduce stress and anxiety. Additionally, yoga can be a helpful tool for promoting healthy circulation and hormonal balance.

It is important to listen to your body during your period and modify your yoga practice as needed. Avoiding inverted postures such as headstands and shoulder stands during menstruation is a common recommendation, as these postures can disrupt the natural flow of blood and increase discomfort. However, each person's experience of menstruation is unique, and what feels comfortable and beneficial for one person may not be the same for another.

Ultimately, the decision to practice yoga during your period is a personal one and should be based on your own comfort level and physical needs. It is always recommended to consult with your healthcare provider if you have any concerns about practicing yoga or other forms of exercise during your period.

Chapter 11:

Yoga is for Everyone, Regardless of Age

Yoga is a practice that has been around for thousands of years, and it is often associated with younger people who are able to perform advanced poses and challenging sequences. However, the truth is that yoga is not just for younger people – it can be enjoyed and practiced by individuals of all ages and levels of experience.

One of the great things about yoga is that it can be modified and adapted to suit the needs of each individual practitioner. For example, older individuals or those with physical limitations or injuries may need to modify certain poses or sequences to ensure that they are safe and appropriate for their bodies. This can involve using props such as blocks, blankets, or straps to support the body and provide additional stability during certain poses.

In fact, many older adults find that practicing yoga can help to improve their overall health and well-being. As we age, our bodies naturally become less flexible and our joints may become stiffer, which can make it difficult to perform certain physical activities. However, regular yoga practice can help to improve flexibility, balance, and mobility, which can help to prevent falls and other injuries in older adults.

Another benefit of yoga for older individuals is that it can help to reduce stress and promote relaxation. Stress is a common issue that affects people of all ages, but it can be particularly challenging for older individuals who may be dealing with health issues, financial concerns, or other life changes. Yoga incorporates breathing exercises and meditation techniques that can help to calm the mind and reduce feelings of anxiety or stress.

In addition to physical and mental benefits, yoga can also provide a sense of community and social connection for older individuals. Many yoga classes are designed specifically for seniors or individuals with mobility limitations, which can provide an opportunity to connect with others who are dealing with similar challenges. This can be especially valuable for older adults who may be experiencing feelings of isolation or loneliness.

Of course, it's important to remember that practicing yoga at any age requires proper instruction and guidance from a qualified teacher. This is especially true for older individuals or those with physical limitations or injuries, who may need additional support and modifications to ensure that they are practicing safely and effectively.

In conclusion, while yoga is often associated with younger people, it is a practice that can benefit individuals of all ages and levels of experience. Whether you are an older adult looking to improve your flexibility and mobility, or a younger person seeking to reduce stress and anxiety, yoga can be an effective tool for improving your physical and mental well-being. So, don't let age hold you back – give yoga a try and see how it can benefit you!

Chapter 12:

Changing Your Food Habits for Yoga

Yoga and diet are often associated with each other, and it is true that practicing yoga can lead to changes in one's eating habits. However, this doesn't mean that you have to make drastic changes in your diet to practice yoga. Rather, it is about making small adjustments that will complement your yoga practice and enhance your overall health and well-being.

Here are some tips for making dietary changes that will support your yoga practice:

1. Eat Whole Foods: Focus on eating a balanced and nutritious diet that includes plenty of wholes, unprocessed foods such as fruits, vegetables, whole grains, and lean proteins. Avoid processed and packaged foods that are high in salt, sugar, and unhealthy fats.
2. Stay Hydrated: Drinking enough water is crucial for overall health, and it's especially important when practicing yoga. Aim to drink at least eight glasses of water a day, and more if you are practicing yoga in a heated room.
3. Eat Light Before Practice: It's best to practice yoga on an empty stomach, but if you must eat before a class, choose light, easily digestible foods such as fruits, vegetables, or a small number of nuts or seeds.
4. Avoid Overeating: Overeating can lead to discomfort and sluggishness, making it difficult to practice yoga. Instead, eat smaller, more frequent meals throughout the day to maintain energy levels and prevent overeating.

5. Listen to Your Body: Pay attention to how your body feels after eating certain foods. If you notice that certain foods make you feel sluggish or uncomfortable, try to avoid them. Similarly, if you find that certain foods give you more energy and make you feel better overall, try to include them more in your diet.

6. Don't Be Too Hard on Yourself: Remember that making dietary changes takes time and effort, and it's okay to slip up sometimes. Don't be too hard on yourself if you indulge in unhealthy foods occasionally, but aim to make healthy choices most of the time.

In summary, making dietary changes to support your yoga practice doesn't have to be difficult or complicated. Simply focus on eating a balanced, nutritious diet, staying hydrated, and listening to your body's needs. By doing so, you can enhance the benefits of your yoga practice and improve your overall health and well-being.

Chapter 13:

The Role of Yoga Teachers as Health Advisors

Yoga is not just about physical postures or asanas. It is a holistic practice that promotes physical, mental, and spiritual well-being. As such, yoga teachers play a crucial role in guiding and supporting their students to achieve their health goals. In this article, we will explore the various ways in which yoga teachers serve as health advisors.

First and foremost, yoga teachers are trained to assess their student's physical abilities and limitations. Before starting a class, yoga teachers typically ask students about any injuries or health conditions they may have. This information helps teachers modify the poses and sequences to suit the student's individual needs. Yoga teachers may also recommend modifications for students who are pregnant or have specific health concerns, such as high blood pressure or arthritis.

In addition to modifying poses, yoga teachers also provide guidance on proper alignment and technique. Correct alignment not only helps students avoid injury but also ensures that they receive the maximum benefits from each pose. Yoga teachers also teach students how to breathe correctly, as breathing is an essential component of the practice. Breathing techniques, such as Ujjayi breath or Pranayama, help students relax, reduce stress, and increase their lung capacity.

Yoga teachers also promote a healthy lifestyle beyond physical practice. They encourage students to adopt a balanced diet, get enough sleep, and manage their stress levels. Many yoga teachers also offer guidance on meditation, mindfulness, and other practices that promote mental and emotional well-being. In this way, yoga teachers serve as health advisors who help their students make lifestyle changes that can have a positive impact on their overall health.

Moreover, yoga teachers are trained to identify imbalances in their students' bodies and minds. They can help students address these imbalances through targeted practices, such as poses that stretch or strengthen specific muscle groups, or through breathing techniques that calm or energize the mind. Yoga teachers may also suggest other complementary practices, such as acupuncture or massage therapy, to help students address specific health concerns.

In addition to one-on-one sessions, many yoga teachers offer workshops and classes that focus on specific health concerns. For example, a yoga teacher might offer a workshop on managing stress or a class for students with back pain. These specialized classes provide students with targeted instruction and support for their specific health needs.

Yoga teachers may also work closely with other health professionals, such as physical therapists or nutritionists, to provide integrated care for their students. For example, a yoga teacher might recommend specific poses or breathing techniques to a student recovering from an injury, while also working with a physical therapist to develop a more comprehensive rehabilitation plan.

Yoga teachers are health advisors who play a vital role in guiding and supporting their students' health and well-being. Through their training and expertise, yoga teachers can help students modify poses, improve alignment, breathe more effectively, and adopt healthy lifestyle habits. They can also help students address specific health concerns, such as injuries or imbalances, and work closely with other health professionals to provide integrated care. As such, yoga teachers are an essential part of any holistic healthcare team.

Chapter 14:

Yoga is Not Just for the Rich

This is a common misconception about yoga that prevents many people from even considering trying it. However, the reality is that yoga is accessible to people of all income levels. While it's true that some yoga classes and retreats can be expensive, there are many affordable options available.

First and foremost, it's important to note that yoga can be practiced at home for free or at a very low cost. There are countless free online resources such as YouTube videos, mobile apps, and websites that provide detailed instructions for practicing yoga at home. All that is required is a yoga mat, which can be purchased for as little as $10. Many community centers, libraries, and parks offer free or low-cost yoga classes.

For those who prefer a more structured environment or enjoy the community aspect of practicing yoga in a group setting, there are many affordable options as well. Many yoga studios offer sliding scale or donation-based classes, which means that students can pay what they can afford. Some studios also offer work-trade opportunities, where students can volunteer in exchange for free or discounted classes.

Another affordable option is to attend yoga classes at a gym or fitness center. Many gyms include yoga classes as part of their membership package, and some even offer free yoga classes to non-members as a way to entice new customers.

It's also worth noting that yoga is not just about attending classes or retreats. It's a lifestyle that can be integrated into everyday life. Practicing yoga doesn't require expensive gear or clothing; comfortable clothes that allow for movement and a quiet space to practice are all needed. Yoga can be practiced outdoors in nature or indoors in a small space.

In addition to physical practice, there are many other aspects of yoga such as meditation, breathing exercises, and philosophy that can be practiced for free or at a low cost. Many meditation and mindfulness apps offer free or low-cost subscriptions, and there are numerous books and online resources available on yoga philosophy and the spiritual aspects of yoga.

Furthermore, yoga is not just a physical practice, but a way of life that can positively impact mental and emotional well-being. It can help reduce stress, anxiety, and depression, and improve overall mental health. The benefits of practicing yoga extend far beyond the physical practice and can be experienced by anyone regardless of income level.

In conclusion, while some aspects of the yoga industry may cater to the affluent, yoga it is accessible to people of all income levels. With free resources available online and affordable options at community centers, gyms, and donation-based yoga studios, anyone can practice yoga regardless of their financial situation. Additionally, the benefits of yoga extend far beyond the physical practice and can have a positive impact on mental and emotional well-being.

Chapter 15:

Yoga is more Than Just a Gentle Exercise

Yoga is often perceived as a gentle exercise, suitable for individuals who are not very active or looking for a low-impact workout. While yoga can indeed be gentle and suitable for beginners, it is also a challenging and dynamic practice that can improve strength, flexibility, and overall fitness. The misconception that yoga is just a gentle exercise may stem from the fact that it often emphasizes slow, controlled movements and breathwork, which can create a sense of calm and relaxation. However, many yoga styles and poses require significant physical effort and can challenge even the most experienced practitioners.

One of the reasons yoga is sometimes perceived as gentle is that it emphasizes the mind-body connection and encourages practitioners to move with awareness and intention. Unlike other forms of exercise that may prioritize intensity and speed, yoga emphasizes proper alignment, breathing, and mindful movement. This approach can create a sense of tranquility and help reduce stress and anxiety. However, this does not mean that yoga is not physically challenging.

In fact, many yoga poses require a significant amount of strength, balance, and flexibility. Arm balances, inversions, and challenging standing poses such as Warrior III or Half Moon require not only physical strength but also mental focus and determination. Additionally, some yoga styles such as Ashtanga or Power Yoga are quite dynamic and can elevate the heart rate, providing a cardiovascular workout that can improve overall fitness.

Another misconception about yoga is that it is not suitable for individuals looking to build muscle or lose weight. While yoga may not provide the same level of calorie burn as high-intensity workouts such as running or weightlifting, it can still be an effective tool for weight management and muscle toning. Yoga poses such as Plank, Chaturanga, and Upward Dog engage the core, arms, and shoulders, while standing poses such as Chair, Crescent Lunge, and Warrior II engage the legs and glutes. Over time, consistent yoga practice can improve muscle strength, tone, and definition.

It is worth noting that not all yoga classes are created equal, and some may indeed be gentler than others. Restorative or Yin Yoga, for example, focus on long holds and passive stretching, making them suitable for individuals recovering from injury or looking for a more meditative practice. However, even in these gentler classes, practitioners can still experience the physical benefits of yoga, such as improved flexibility and joint mobility.

In conclusion, while yoga may emphasize the mind-body connection and encourage practitioners to move with awareness and intention, it is not just a gentle exercise. Yoga can be challenging and dynamic, improving strength, flexibility, and overall fitness. Whether you are a beginner or an experienced practitioner, there is a yoga style and practice suitable for your needs and goals.

Conclusion

Practicing yoga is not just about physical exercise, but also a holistic approach to mental, emotional, and spiritual well-being. Through regular practice, one can cultivate mindfulness, reduce stress and anxiety, increase flexibility, strength, and balance, and promote overall health and wellness.

There are various styles of yoga to choose from, each with its own unique benefits and challenges. It is important to find a style and teacher that resonates with your needs and goals and to approach your practice with an open and non-judgmental mindset.

Yoga is not just for the young or the flexible, but for anyone willing to explore and commit to the practice. Modifications and props can be used to adapt poses to individual needs and abilities.

Lastly, yoga is not just a physical exercise but a way of life. The principles of yoga, such as ahimsa (non-harming), Satya (truthfulness), and svadhyaya (self-study), can be applied to all aspects of life, promoting greater awareness and compassion towards oneself and others.

Whether you are new to yoga or have been practicing for years, may your journey be one of self-discovery, growth, and transformation. Namaste.